Mighty Me

A Magical Journey of Courage, Love, and Strength

written by

ANALY NAVARRO

illustrated by

CITLALI GARDUÑO

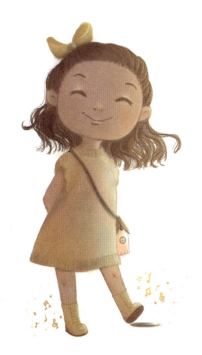

*Stay Mighty,
Analy N.*

Copyright © 2021 Analy Navarro

All rights reserved. No portion of this book may be reproduced in any form without permission from the publisher, except as permitted by U.S. copyright law.

Text: Analy Navarro
Book cover & illustrations: Citlali Garduño

For permissions contact: AnalyNav@me.com

ISBN: 978-0-578-91896-9

To my Mighty Julia, who continues to amaze us every day with her love, strength, and magic. You are amazing.

To all the mighty children who traveled on their own magical quest to find their gift of life and to the amazing parents who were by their side every step of the way.

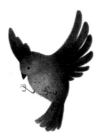

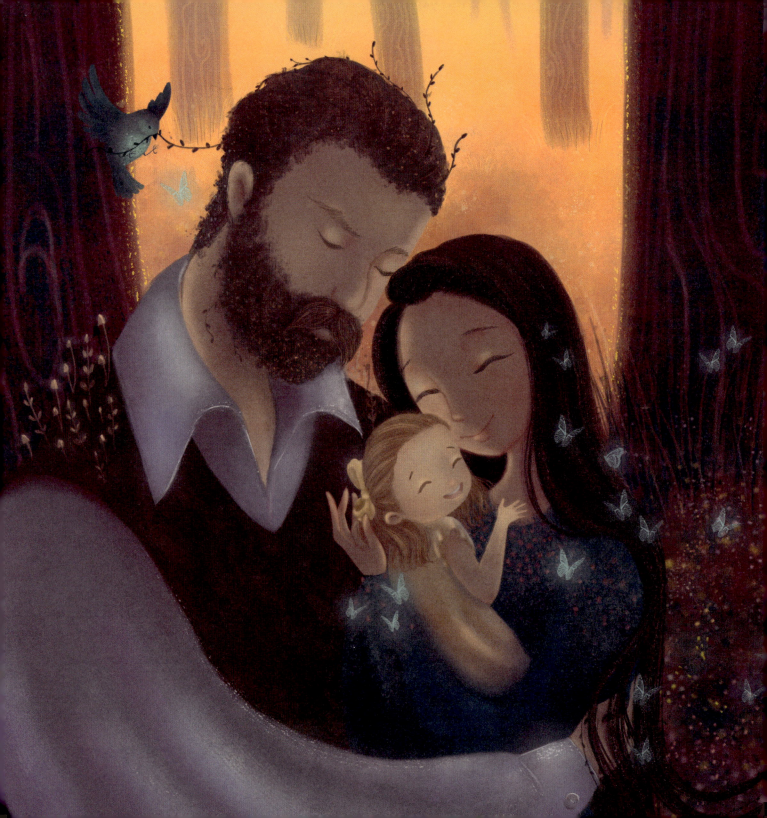

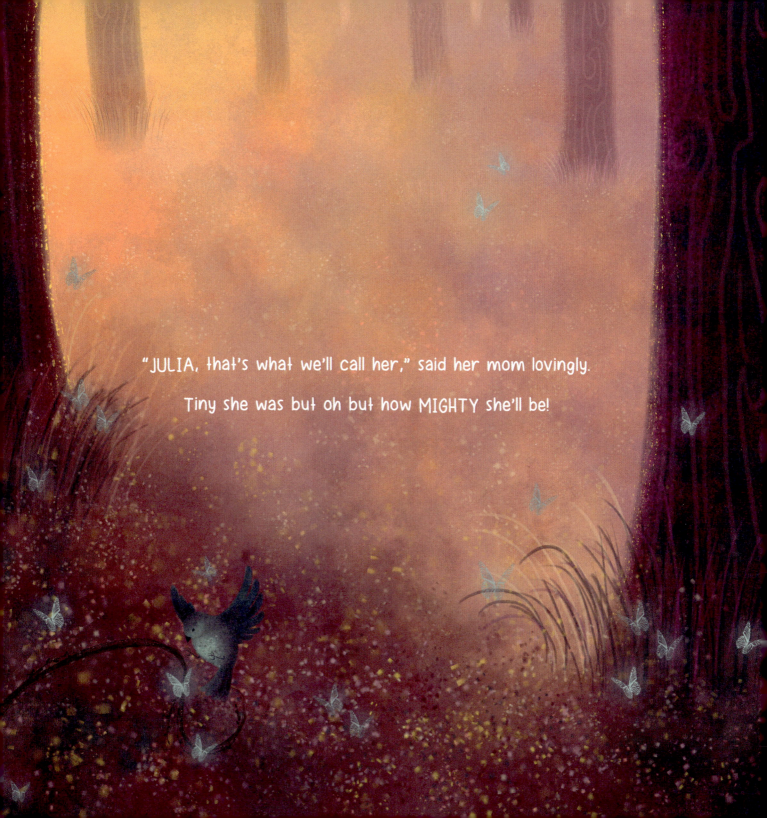

"JULIA, that's what we'll call her," said her mom lovingly.

Tiny she was but oh but how MIGHTY she'll be!

She had CURIOUS eyes, an ITTY-BITTY nose

and HAPPY little dancing toes.

So AMAZING was she that her GREATEST ADVENTURE started

immediately!

And her life depended on it, desperately.

She was FADING AWAY

little by little every day

but so determined was she NOT to DISMAY

that a little thing like this wouldn't get in her way.

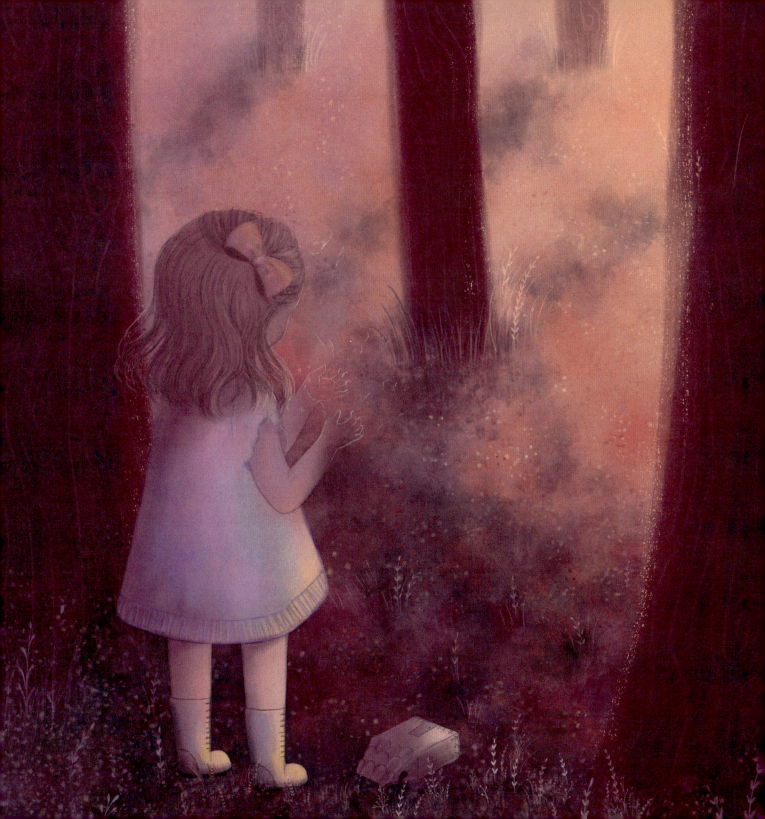

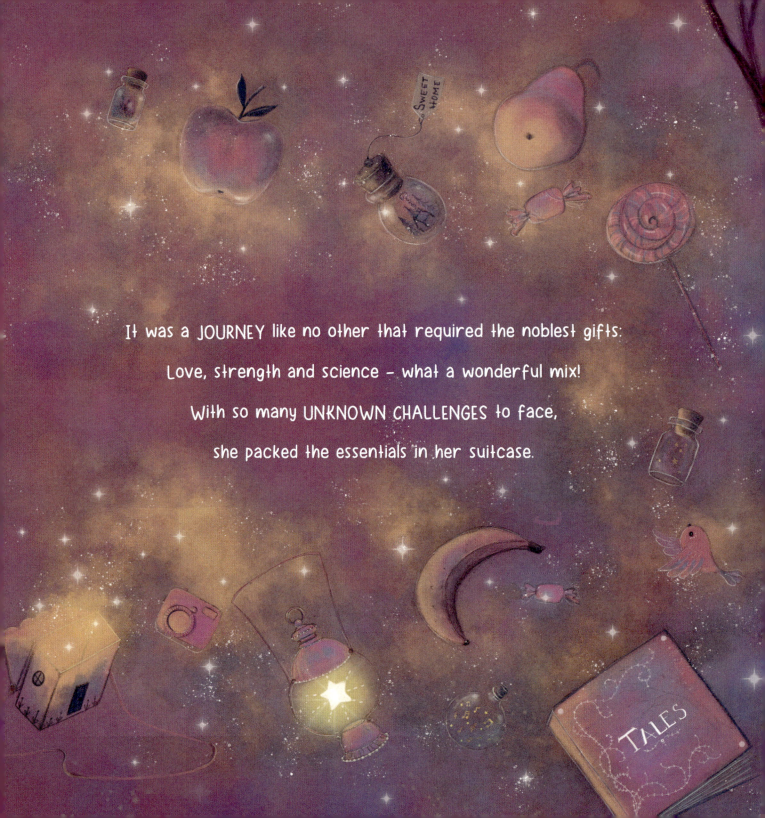

It was a JOURNEY like no other that required the noblest gifts:

Love, strength and science - what a wonderful mix!

With so many UNKNOWN CHALLENGES to face,

she packed the essentials in her suitcase.

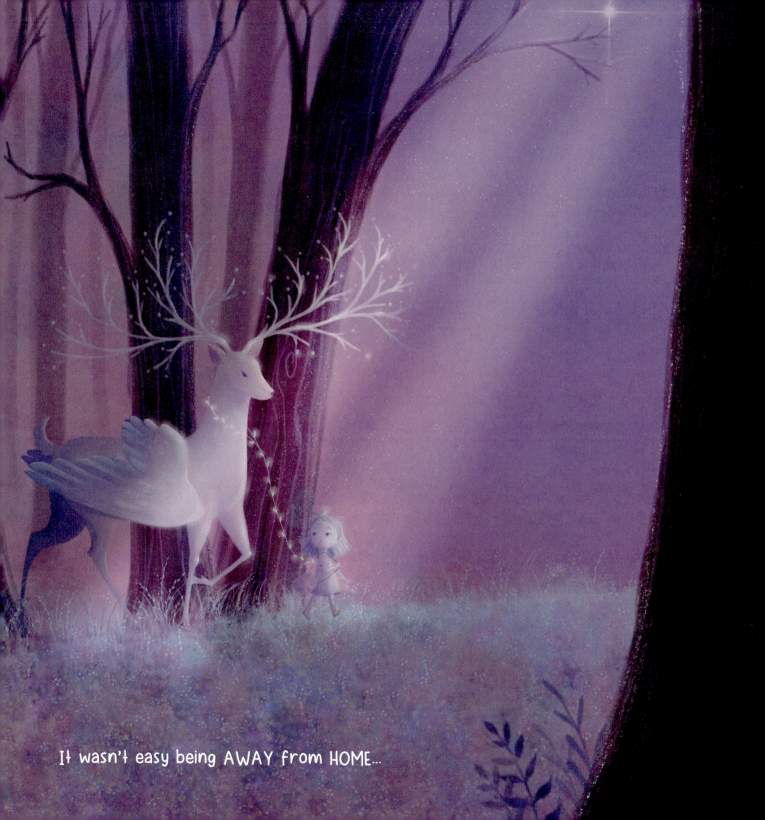

It wasn't easy being AWAY from HOME...

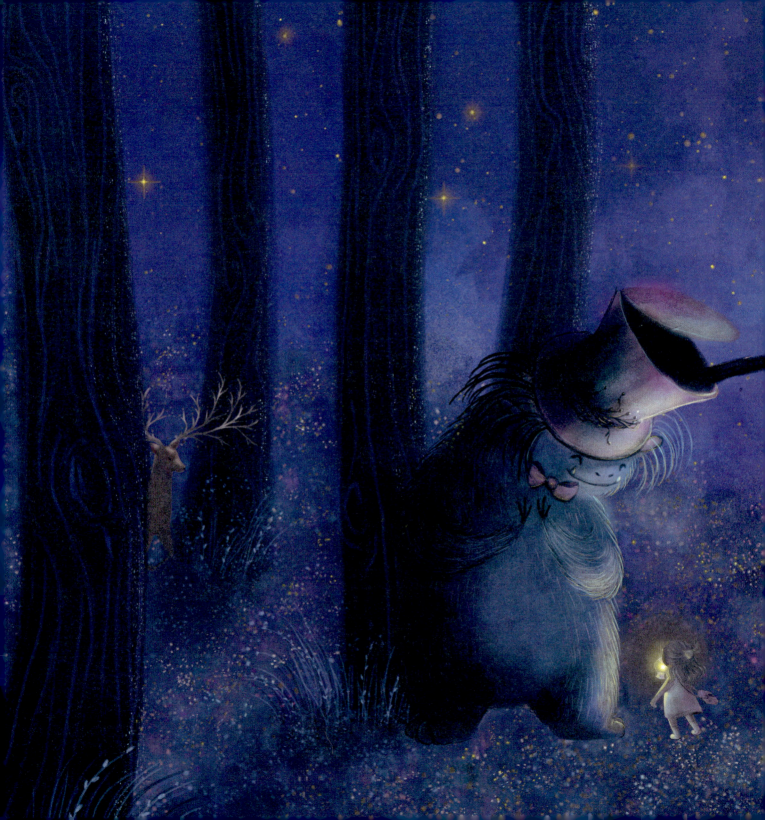

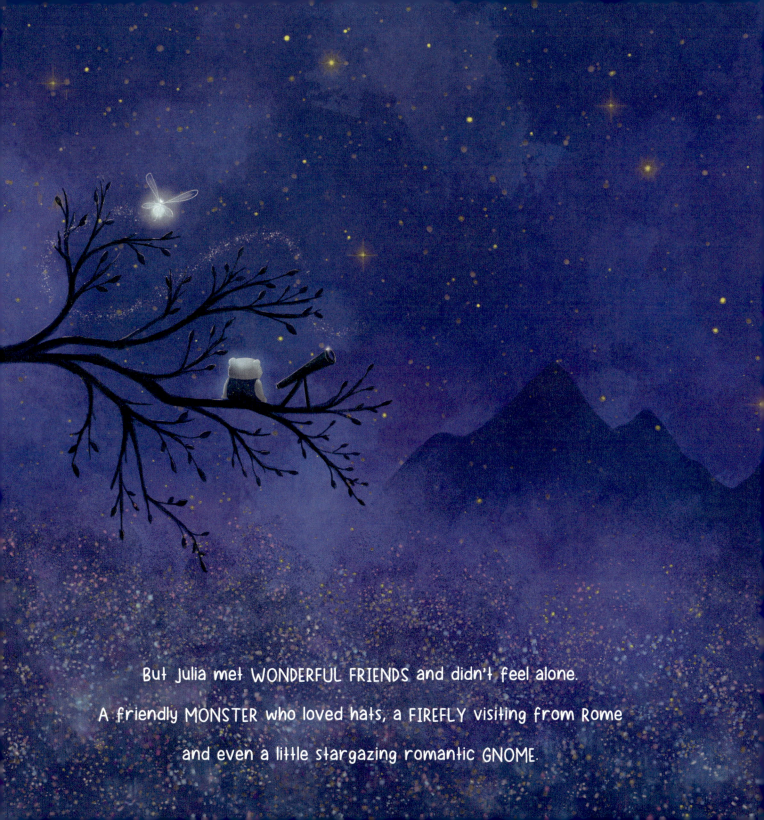

But Julia met WONDERFUL FRIENDS and didn't feel alone.

A friendly MONSTER who loved hats, a FIREFLY visiting from Rome

and even a little stargazing romantic GNOME.

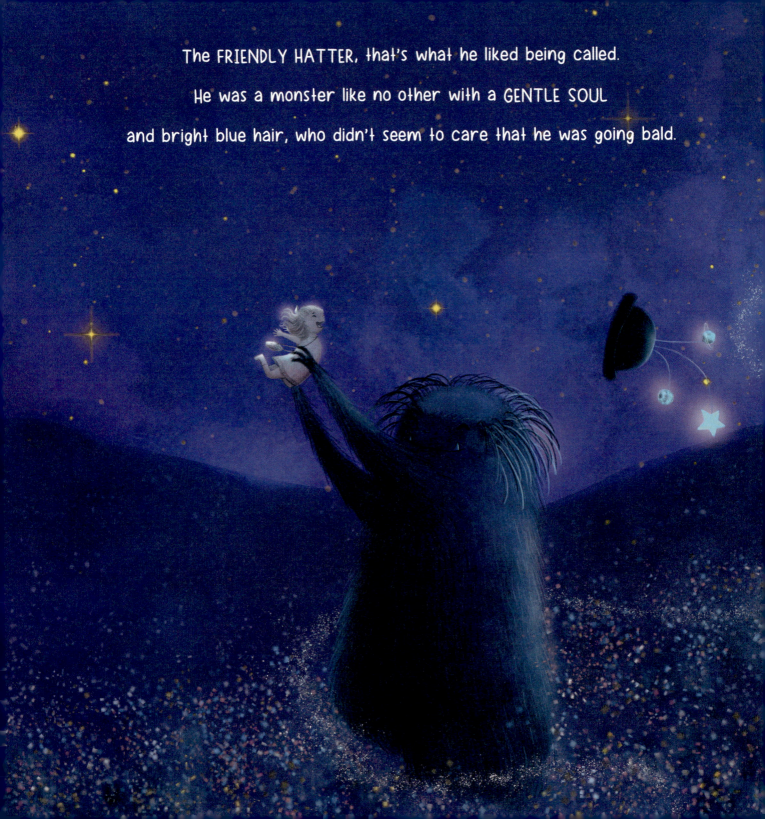

The FRIENDLY HATTER, that's what he liked being called.

He was a monster like no other with a GENTLE SOUL

and bright blue hair, who didn't seem to care that he was going bald.

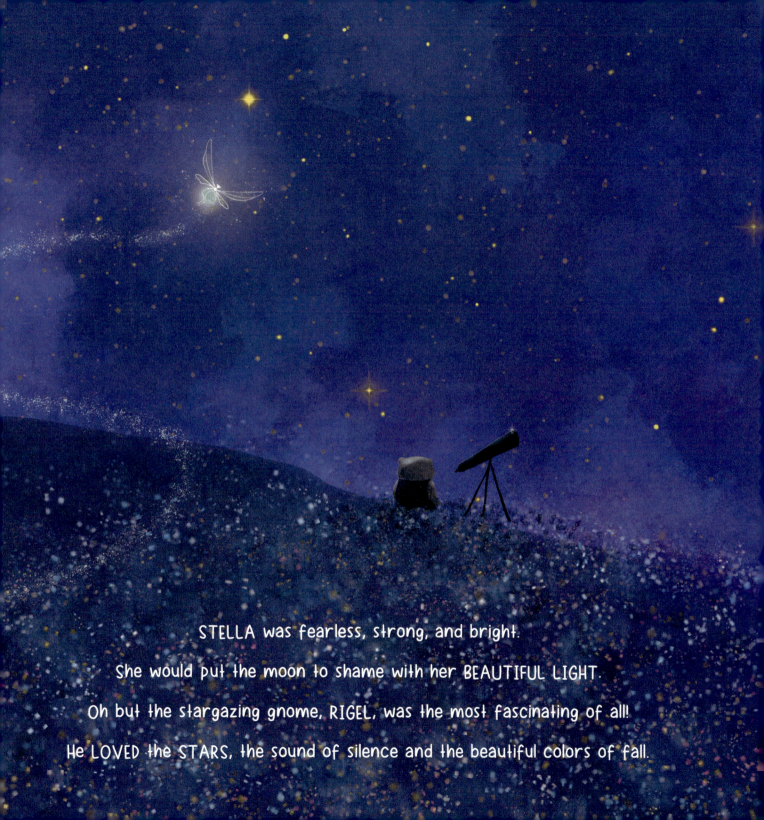

STELLA was fearless, strong, and bright.

She would put the moon to shame with her BEAUTIFUL LIGHT.

Oh but the stargazing gnome, RIGEL, was the most fascinating of all!

He LOVED the STARS, the sound of silence and the beautiful colors of fall.

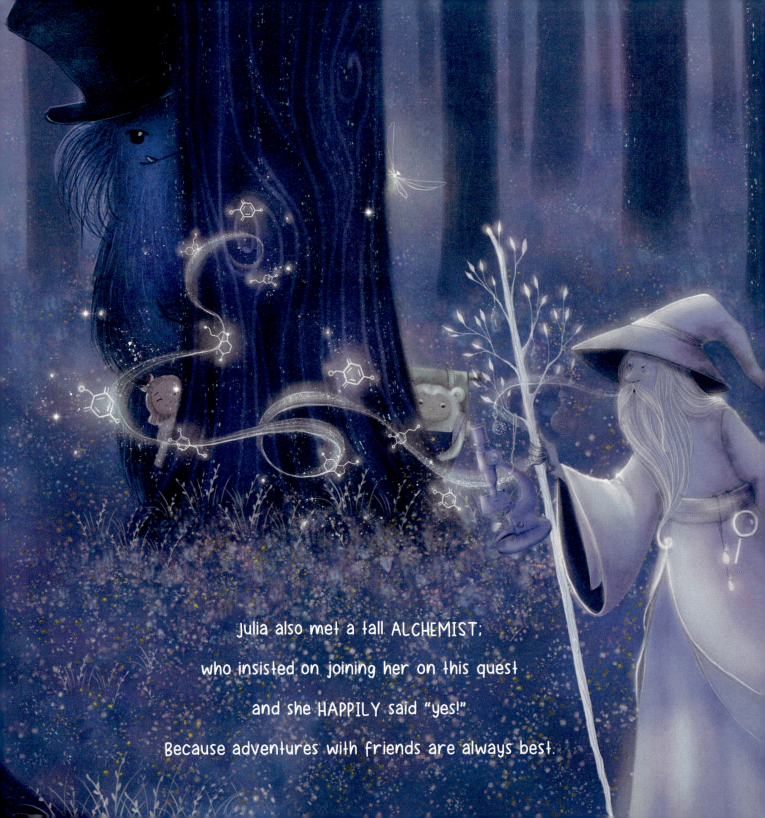

Julia also met a tall ALCHEMIST,

who insisted on joining her on this quest

and she HAPPILY said "yes!"

Because adventures with friends are always best.

What were they SEARCHING FOR, you might ask?

Well, they had quite the task!

They had to FIND a RARE STONE containing the magic of life

and it had to be the perfect match in COLOR and SIZE.

JULIA was so glad that the ALCHEMIST came along,

with his knowledge and science he helped her stay

healthy and strong.

His specialty was helping kids find their MAGICAL STONE

and he could transform any metal into gold with a formula of his own.

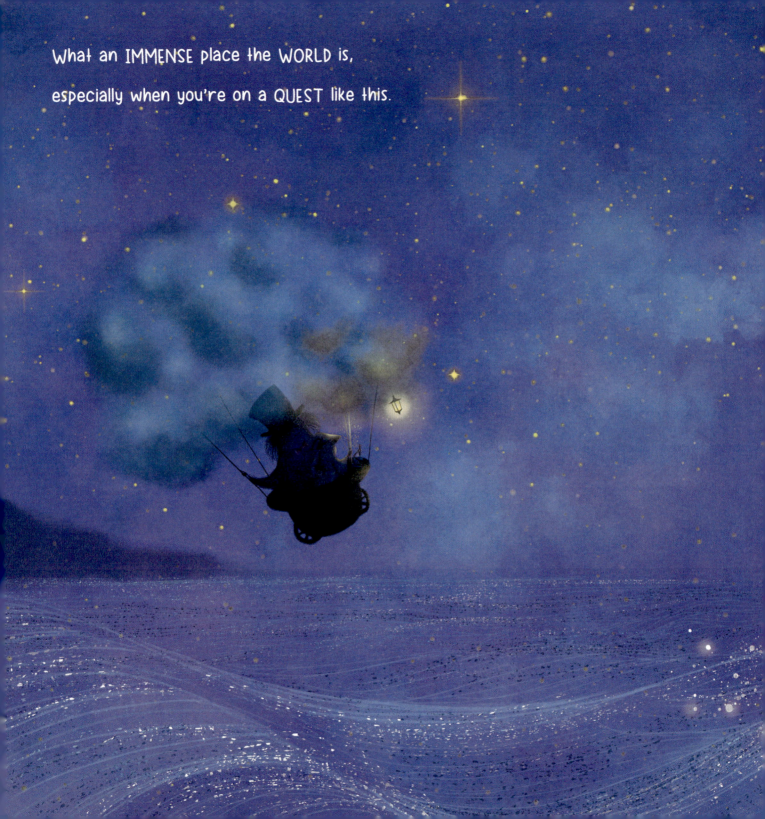

What an IMMENSE place the WORLD is, especially when you're on a QUEST like this.

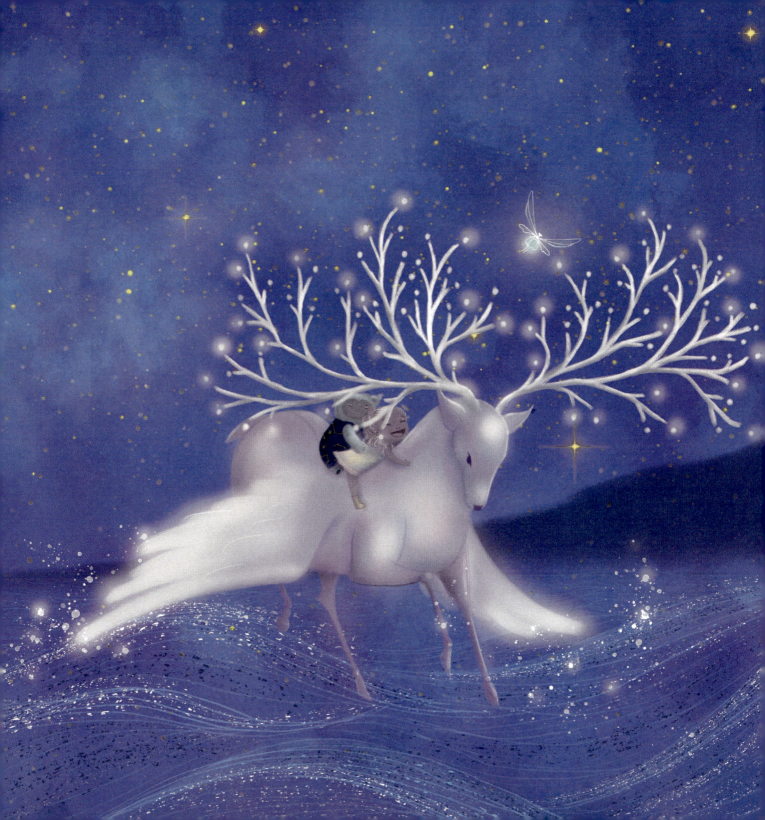

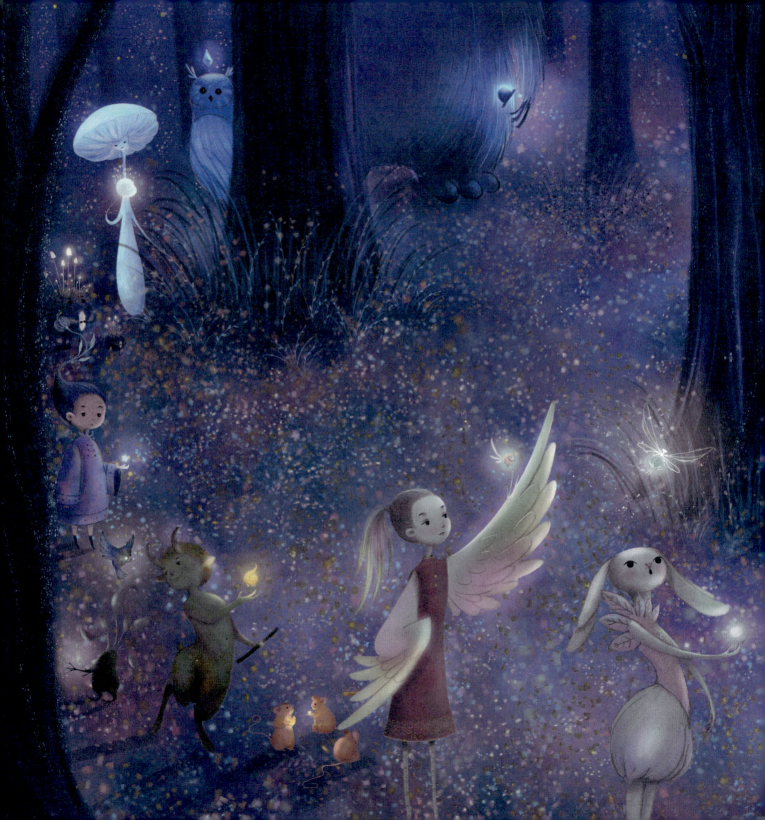

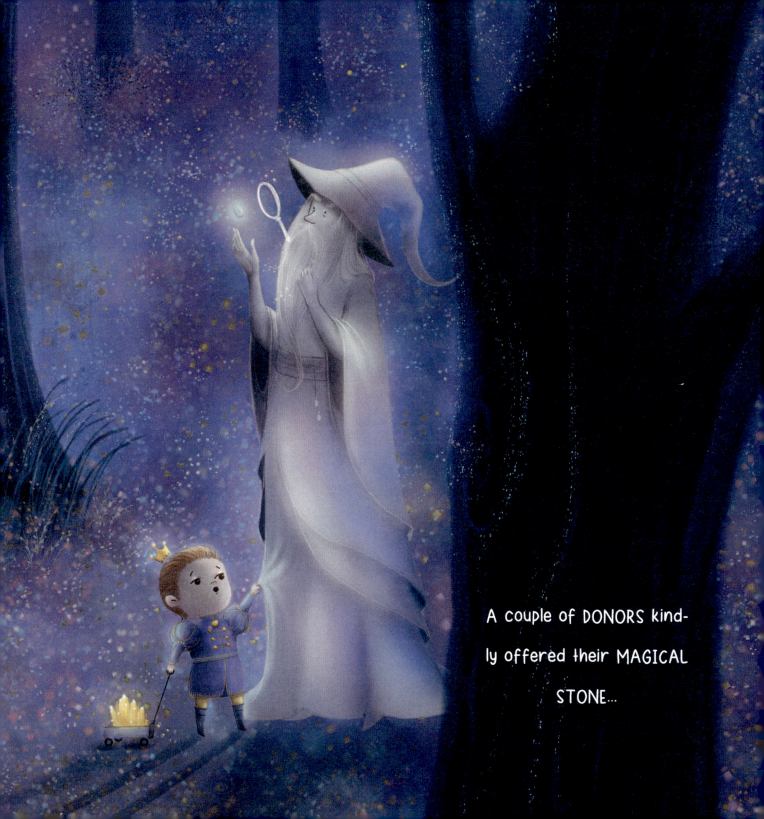

A couple of DONORS kindly offered their MAGICAL STONE...

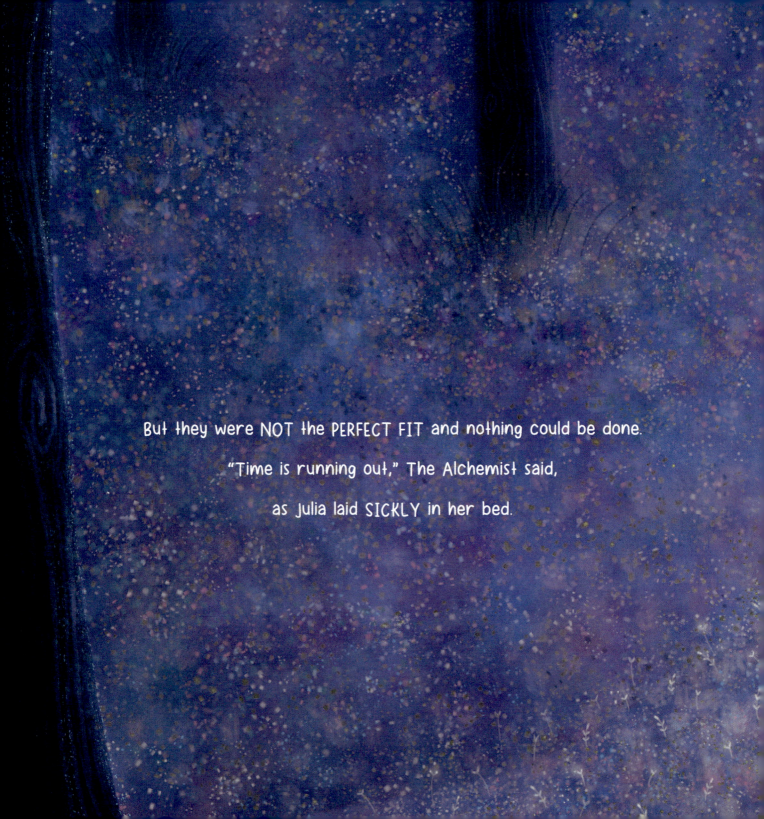

But they were NOT the PERFECT FIT and nothing could be done.

"Time is running out," The Alchemist said,

as Julia laid SICKLY in her bed.

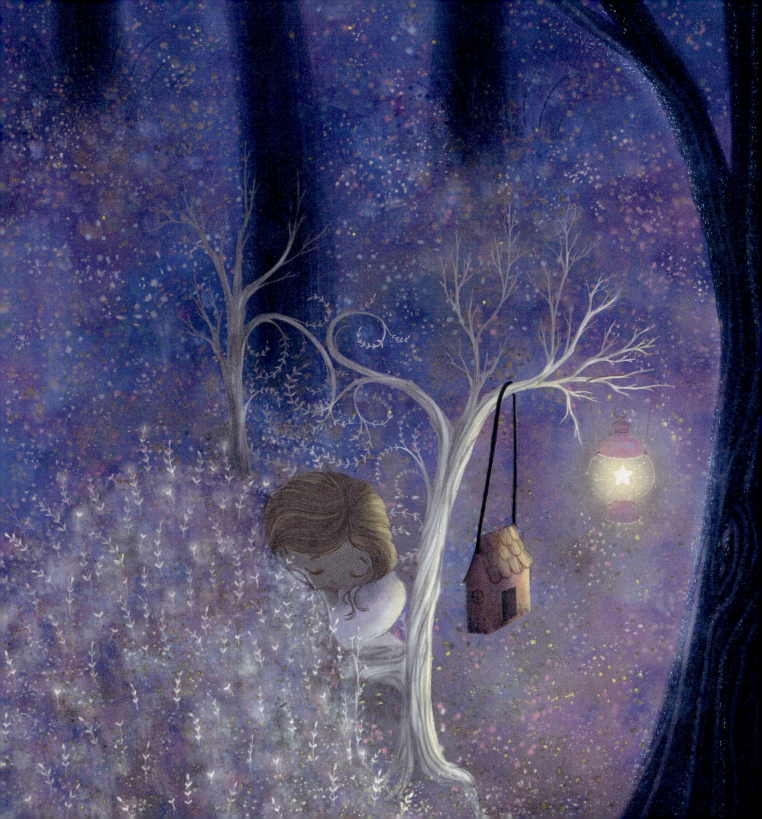

"We volunteer," said her MOM and DAD,

"Take MY STONE and GIVE HER a small part.

But could that be done?"

"Well," replied the Alchemist, "NOTHING is IMPOSSIBLE

under the sun!"

Along with some friends,

the Alchemist got to work on the magical stone,

such an IMPORTANT TASK couldn't be done alone.

They carefully weighed and measured both stones,

it took them hours to check for color and tone.

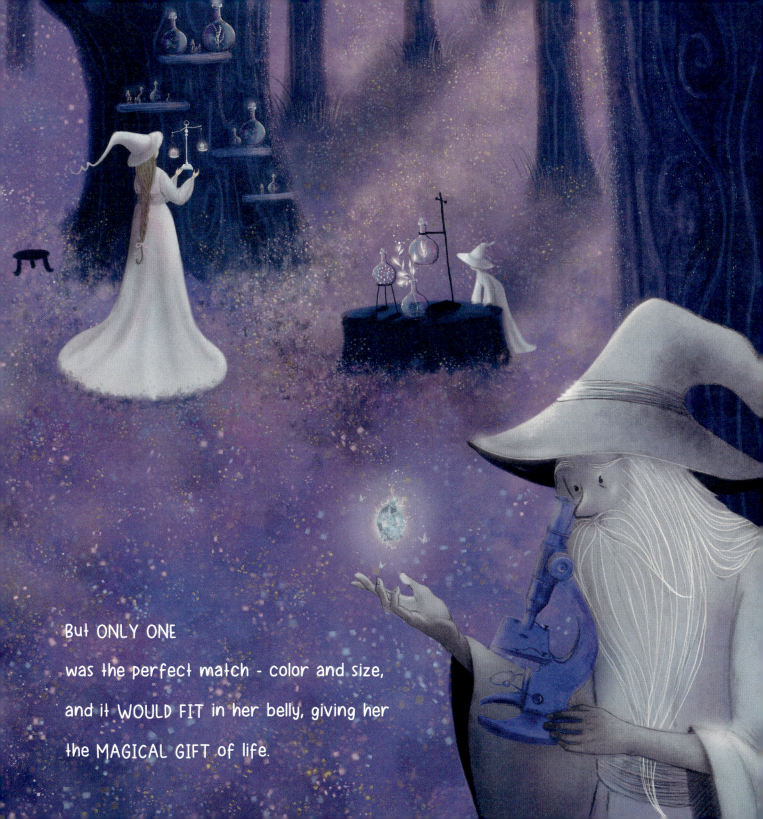

But ONLY ONE
was the perfect match - color and size,
and it WOULD FIT in her belly, giving her
the MAGICAL GIFT of life.

The INTRICATE PROCEDURE took them a very long time,
and all the work was worth it because the outcome was BEYOND SUBLIME!

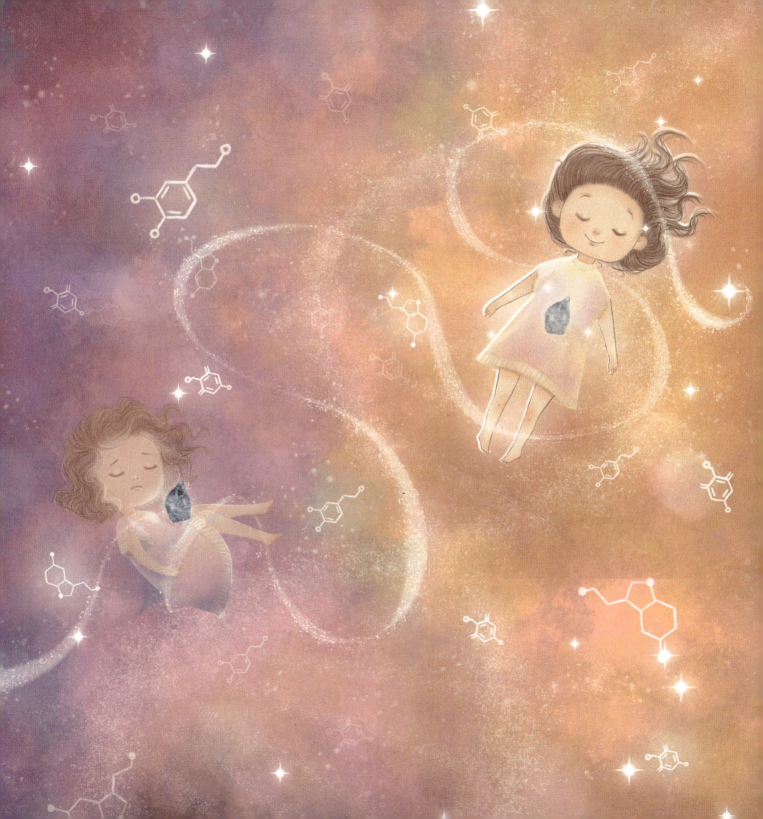

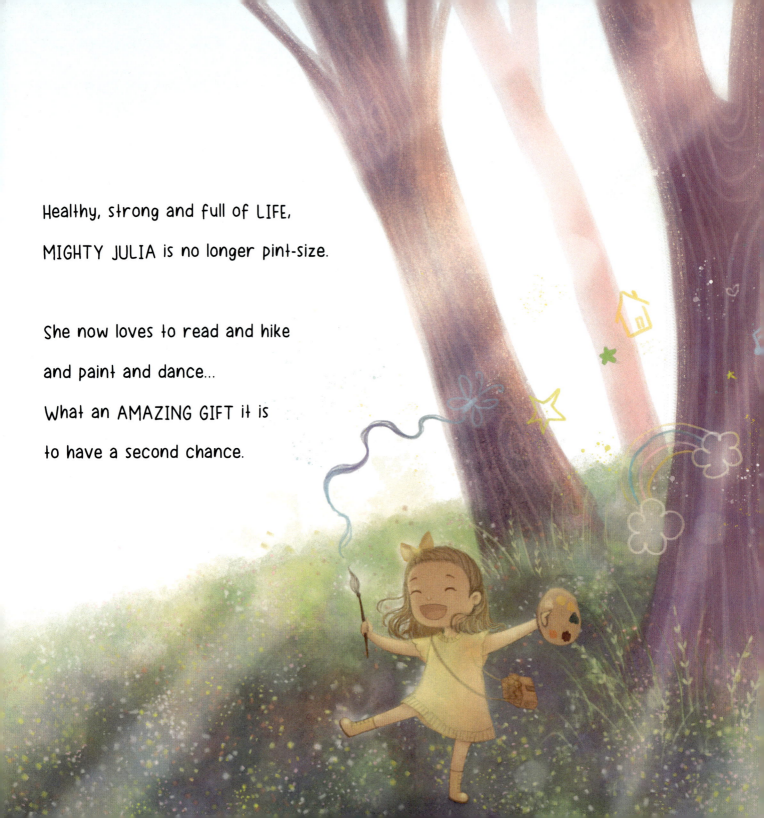

Healthy, strong and full of LIFE,
MIGHTY JULIA is no longer pint-size.

She now loves to read and hike
and paint and dance...
What an AMAZING GIFT it is
to have a second chance.

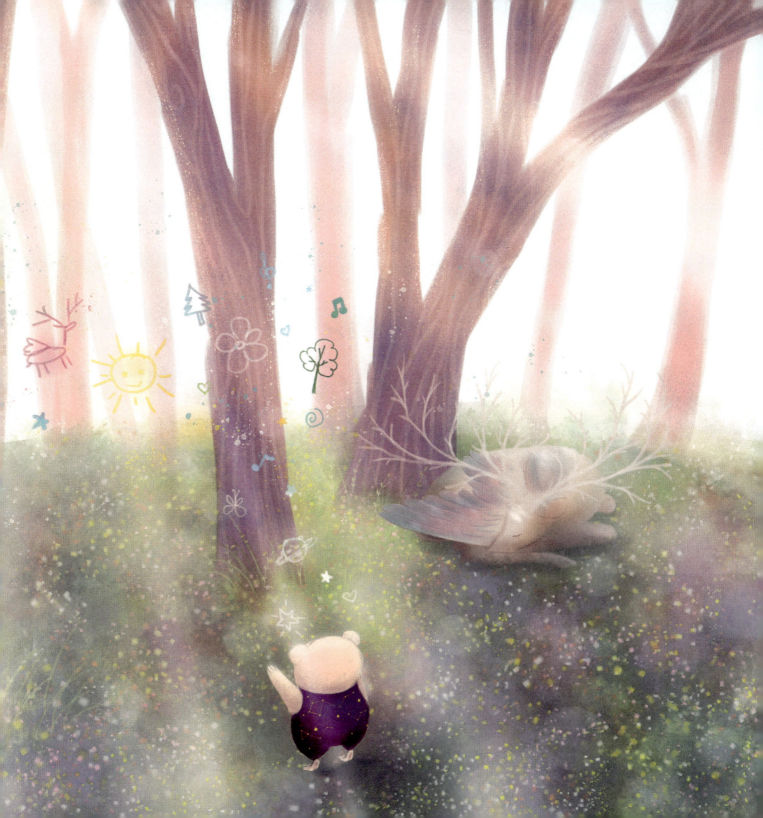

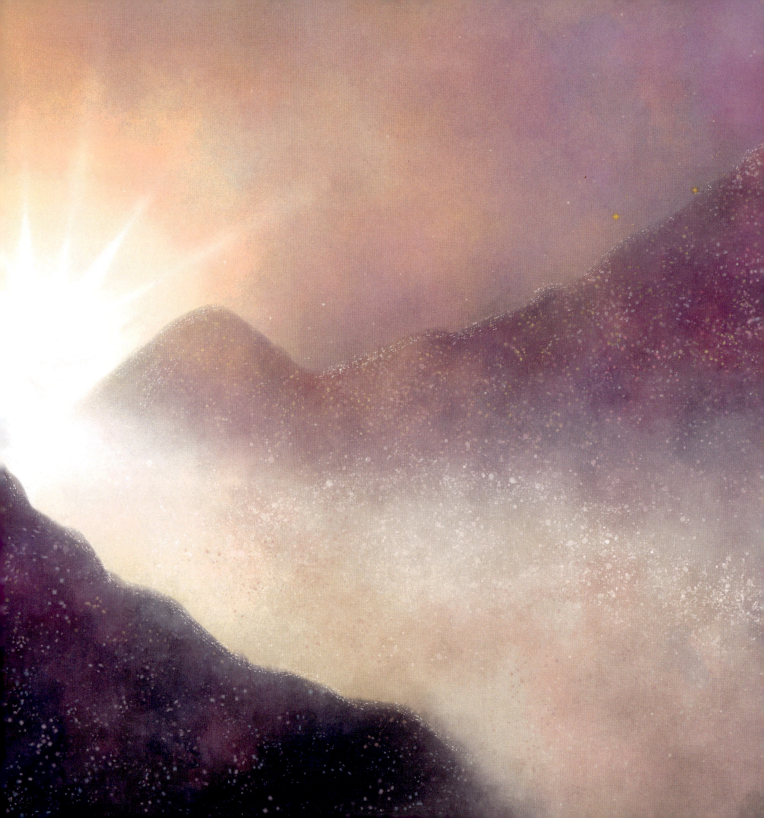

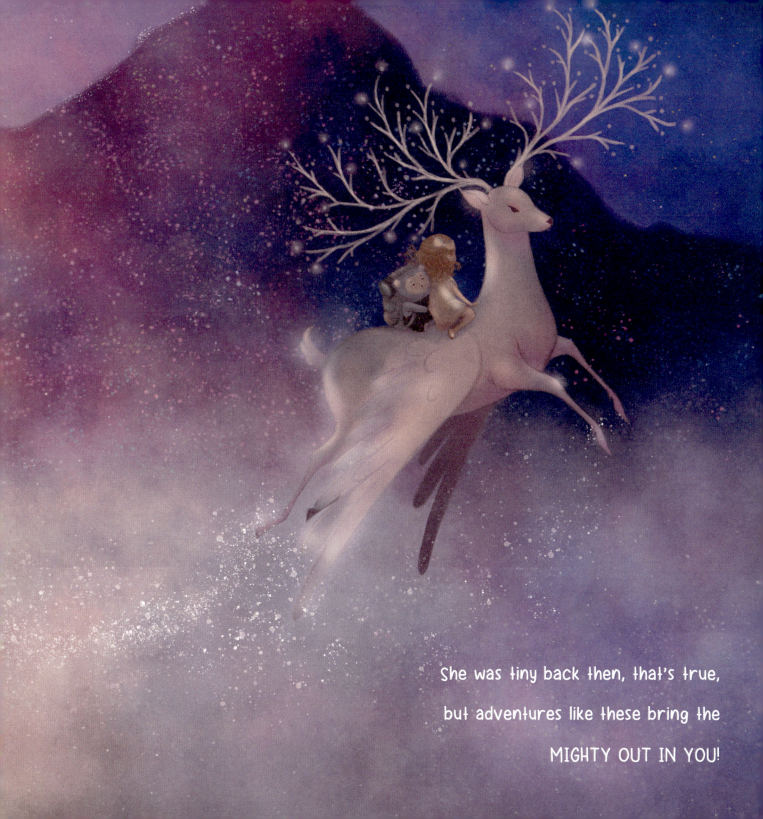

She was tiny back then, that's true,

but adventures like these bring the

MIGHTY OUT IN YOU!

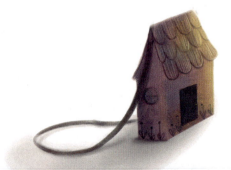

Made in the USA
Columbia, SC
13 July 2021

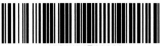